An Every Day
Guide to
Pancha Karma

Vaidya Varsha Galgali

Kashyapa Fisher

Copyright © 2018 The Arogya Center
All rights reserved.
ISBN: 1718934092
ISBN 13: 9781718934092

INVOCATION

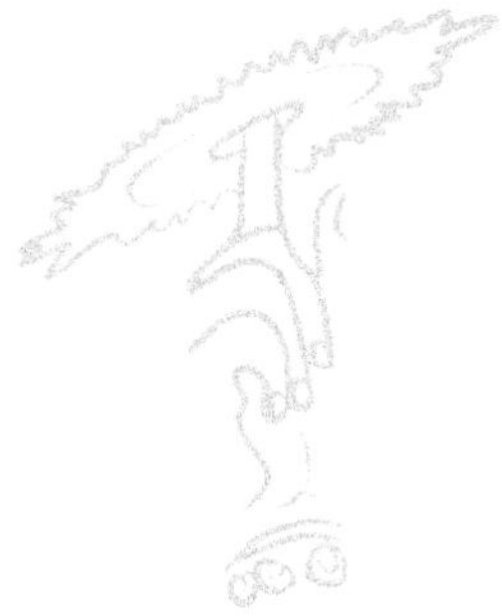

अदविद्याय वदिमाहे अरोग्य नुग्रहाय धीमाहि
तन्नो धन्वन्तरि पुरच्छोधायत्

The humble efforts of a limited individual or even a group of
dedicated people beholden of the same aim and vision may
indeed serve in bringing forth a bountiful harvest of
knowledge, beauty and utility- but it is ever Grace alone that
is truly the deciding factor. Such Grace is the magic that
causes the seed to sprout, the sun to shine, the wind to blow,
the breath to breathe, the heart to open and love to unfold.
Before the mysterious and ineffable source of that Grace, we
bow down and offer up these small efforts of ours.

लोकाः समस्तः सुखिनो भवन्तु

May All Beings be Happy and Healthy

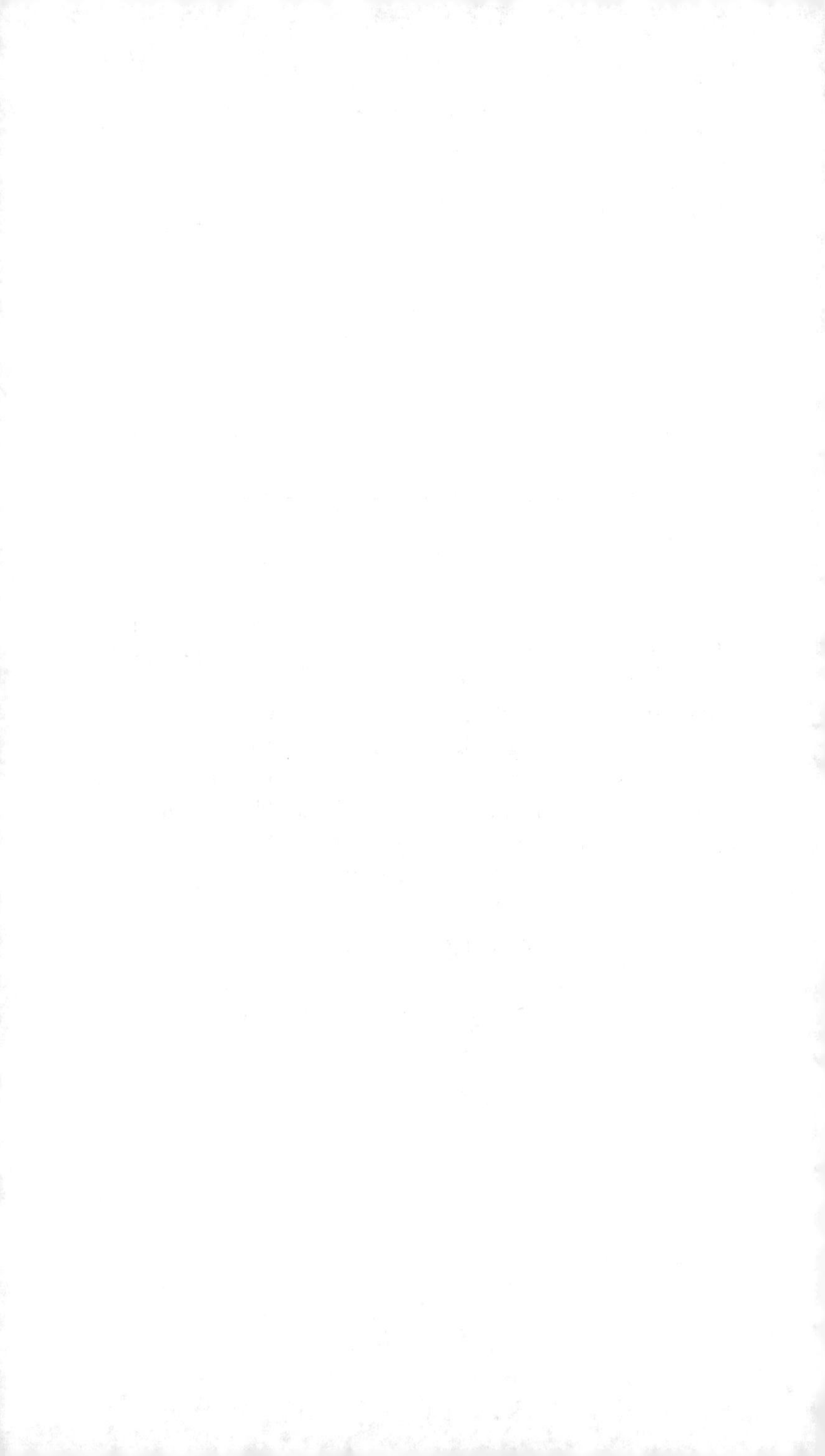

Contents

Introduction

For countless thousands of years, the techniques and methods of what is now popularly termed as 'Pancha Karma' have been utilized by skilled Ayurvedic Physicians to eradicate disease and to restore health and vitality to humanity. These practices are deeply rooted in the ancient texts of Ayurveda,[1] some of the oldest of which, such as the Charaka Samhita and Sushruta Samhita, were recorded around 1500 BC, nearly five thousand years ago. Pancha Karma, properly speaking, is not a singular noun denoting a particular thing or a standard treatment sequence. Rather, Pancha Karma in fact describes Pancha Karmas: Five Therapeutic Procedures used to remove obstructions.

Pancha means 'Five' and Karma means 'Curative Action,' 'Procedure,' 'Treatment.' To be more precise, the Pancha Karmas refer to five 'Shodhana Karmas,' actions which are 'purifying' or 'deeply cleansing,' 'which remove obstruction.' These Shodhana actions have the specific aim of purifying or removing Doshas,[2] the bodily humors. This term Dosha is utilized in Ayurveda to describe the fundamental physiological programming forces of the body. When functioning properly and harmoniously, the Doshas are the cause of health and longevity. When functioning abnormally, the same Doshas vitiate the body's tissues and critical processes, causing disease and physiological disorder.

Through the judicious employment of these five therapeutic procedures, the Pancha Karmas, excessive Doshas, which are the primary cause of disease, are expelled out from the body.

---

[1] Ayurveda, literally 'the Knowledge of Life,' is described in the Charaka Samhita as 'that which describes what is beneficial and detrimental to life and the states of happiness and suffering.'

[2] Dosha, literally 'that which corrupts' or 'spoils'

It is important to note that the Pancha Karmas of Ayurveda stand apart from the 'Cleanses' and 'Detox Regimens' of other healing modalities such as Naturopathy in that while these strive to purify the body of waste products such as metabolites and environmental toxins, the efforts of Ayurveda go a step beyond, simultaneously purifying the body and resetting the physiological forces and programming intelligence of the body which allow for this corruption to transpire in the first place.

Ideally, these procedures should be undergone annually even by healthy persons during the transition between seasons to support optimal health and longevity. As the seasons move from one to the next, the Doshas naturally well up and increase within the body. Thus, by resorting to Pancha Karma treatments at these opportune times eradicate the Doshas before they are able to corrupt the physiological processes of the body and sow the seeds of disease. Proper recourse to these purifying procedures protects the homeostasis of the body, curbs the aging process to support longevity and, under appropriate conditions and with proper application, can assist in the treatment of and recovery from virtually all diseases.

The methods and practices of these Pancha Karmas have flowered forth from Ayurveda in its purity since time immemorial. Within the unique cosmos of Ayurveda's medical system, these therapeutic actions have very specific definitions and aims. Unfortunately, in the modern world, especially in the West, this term 'Pancha Karma' has become corrupted to imply a great many things, while the essence has been lost. Most commonly, Pancha Karma is used to describe different Spa Packages in which one receives daily oil-massages, sauna or sweat box treatments, beautifying treatments, aromatherapy, etc…. In some cases one may also observe a restricted diet, often just Khichari[3], take pacifying herbs and teas and may possibly undergo a mild purgation or receive enemas. These are usually marketed in five, seven or ten day packages.

These Pancha Karma or 'PK' Spa Packages are entirely antithetical to the classical vision and purpose of Ayurveda as a medical system and distort the concept of the Pancha Karmas. While these Spa Packages may well be deeply relaxing and pacifying, which indeed can have great value especially in today's increasingly hectic world, to call these packages as Pancha Karma is misleading and demeans the actual practice of clinical Ayurveda and the vision of the Ancient Sages who have handed this knowledge down from antiquity.

Fundamentally, the authentic and responsible practice of the Pancha Karmas cannot be 'packaged.' These procedures must be precisely tailored to the needs of the Patient, taking into account one's constitution, age, accustomed diet and habits, strength, diseases, the stages and specific expression of those diseases, the environment one lives in, the environment the procedures will be performed in, the season, abnormal weather patterns and numerous other factors. It would be impossible to perform all five of these therapeutic procedures even in a 10-day package and incredibly unlikely that one could responsibly perform even one of the primary purifying procedures in a 5-day package. In many cases a Patient is a candidate for only one of these procedures or perhaps a unique combination of them, or indeed maybe none at all. It is this specific and refined attention to the uniqueness and subjectivity of the Patient and environment and in turn the reflection of this consideration in the formulation of a unique and subjective clinical protocol that gives both Ayurveda and the Pancha Karmas their efficacy, beauty and profound

---

[3] Rice and Lentils cooked together into a homogenous porridge

healing capacity.

The purpose of this work is to elucidate, in brief, what these Pancha Karmas and their required Preparatory Procedures actually are, along with their indications, contraindications and proper administration.

PURVA KARMAS: PREPARATORY PROCEDURES

Before subjecting the body to the more intensive cleansing procedures described as the Pancha Karmas, one must first undergo a series of preparatory procedures to detoxify and give resilience to the tissues and organs of the body. The most important of these preparatory procedures are Oleation and Sudation.

Snehana: Oleation Therapy

In Oleation Therapy, unctuous materials such as oils and animal fats are used to nourish and lubricate the body inside and out, loosen morbid, unwanted materials and to give the body's tissues greater resilience and elasticity. There are two general methods of employing Oleation Therapy: Internally and Externally.

INTERNAL OLEATION THERAPY

Internal Oleation Therapy involves the oral consumption of different fats. These fats could be vegetable oils such as Almond Oil, Coconut Oil and different Herbally-Medicated forms of Sesame Oil or animal fats such as Butter, Tallows or Muscles Fats, Bone Marrow and, most commonly, Ghee-Clarified Butter.

Internal Oleation Therapy can secure a wide variety of health benefits. For this reason, there are Three Forms of Internal Oleation Therapy, each one varying in its method of administration to produce specific aims or benefits. These three forms or methods of Internal Oleation Therapy are Building Oleation Therapy, Pacifying Oleation Therapy and Purifying Oleation Therapy.[4]

Building Internal Oleation Therapy

As the name implies, this method of Internal Oleation Therapy gives bulk and strength, increasing bodily mass and power. Healthy fats, selected appropriately for one's unique constitution and environment, are among the most essential and vital nourishing substances.

To accomplish Building Internal Oleation Therapy, fats are taken in small quantity with food, especially in combination with meats, soups, milk, rice and other dietary staples. This enables these high quality fats to be digested and integrated into the bodily tissues, imbuing the tissues with strength, good moisture, smoothness, resilience and shine. Because this method uses the least amount of fat (in comparison with the other two), it can be employed for extended periods of time to facilitate deep nourishment.

Pacifying Internal Oleation Therapy

 In nature, oily substances are used as a fuel to kindle and ignite fire. The same is true within the body. The intake of good fatty substances kindles and strengthens the digestive fire which in turn gives strength and radiance to the body itself. When this digestive fire is strong and burning brightly, giving strength of immunity, endurance and metabolizing food stuffs into robust and resilient tissues, no disease can afflict the body.

In this method of Internal Oleation, conservative amounts of fats are taken followed by hot water on an empty stomach just before meals when the hunger is strong. This is continued for a prescribed amount of time which can range from weeks to more than a month at a time. This form of Internal

---

[4] In Ayurvedic terminology these three forms of Internal Oleation Therapy are called as 1) Shodhana Snehapan (Purifying), 2) Shamana Snehapan (Pacifying) and 3) Brumhana Snehapan (Building)

Oleation gives strength to the body and digestive fire and can calm and pacify a number of ailments and disorders, most commonly those arising from Vata[5] and Pitta[6] Doshas.

Purifying Internal Oleation Therapy

This is the method of Internal Oleation Therapy that is used specifically to prepare the body for one of the Pancha Karma Procedures. This method lubricates all of the gross and subtle bodily channels so that the Doshas can be dislodged and expelled out from the body. It also imbues great resilience and elasticity to the tissues so that they can easily endure any strain involved in this process of elimination.

In this method, generally only Ghee or Herbally Medicated Vegetable Oils are used. The chosen fat is taken on an empty stomach in the early morning close to sunrise. At this time the digestive tract should have processed all of the food material from the previous day, but, being early, the digestive fire should not yet be burning so brightly as to create strong hunger. It is during this golden window of opportunity that the fatty substance can best spread throughout the body and dislodge the Doshas because it will not encounter any obstacles from food stuffs still being digested and, because the fire isn't yet too strong, the fat itself is spared from being too quickly digested.

After taking the fat, one should avoid eating and drinking

---

[5] Vata Dosha is composed of the Air and Ether Elements. When imbalanced it can produce Wasting, Dark Discolouration, Desire for Warm Things, Tremors, Constipation, Fatigue, Poor Sleep and Sensory Functioning, Excessive Talking and Confusion. -Ashtanga Hrudayam Ch 11:5-6

[6] Pitta Dosha is composed of Fire and Water. When imbalanced it manifests Yellow Discolorations throughout the Body and in the Stool and Urine, Excessive Hunger and Thirst, Burning Sensation and Poor Sleep. -Ashtanga Hrudayam Ch 11:6

until there is a strong and clear sensation of hunger, indicating that the fat from the morning has thoroughly spread through the channels and has been properly digested. Also during this process, it is important to eat and drink only warm food and warm water and also to use only warm water for all daily activities like hand washing, bathing etc…. as cool water and substances constrict the channels of the body which can create complications.

The amounts of the fats given will vary from person to person as per digestive capacity, constitution, age, season and the diseases or symptoms that are being treated. Each day an increasing amount of the fatty substance is given. This process is usually continued for a period of three to seven days and is continued until the body has become thoroughly lubricated. This is evidenced by smooth, easy and clear elimination of gas, bowels and belches and the appearance of oil in the stool. At this point the body is ready for one the Pancha Karma Purifying Procedures.

EXTERNAL OLEATION THERAPY

This External Oleation Therapy is the application of fats and oils to the body, most popularly in the form of Abhyanga or Oil Massage, a treatment which has come to be held as a great signature and herald of Ayurveda.

In Abhyanga, the fats applied to the body are absorbed internally via the pores of the skin which in effect are like so many countless billons of tiny mouths which eat it up, directly nourishing the tissues and pacifying the Doshas. While oils such as Sesame, Sunflower, Almond and Coconut are the most common fats used for Abhyanga because of their availability and economy, Ayurveda utilizes a great plethora of fatty substances individually and in combination for External Oleation Therapy such as Ghee, Animal Fats, Milks, etc…. Especially potent for External Oleation Therapy are the thousands of different Ayurvedic recipes of herbally medicated oils and fats which have been concocted for the wide varieties of constitution, environments and disorders.

Abhyanga is considered an essential observance for the healthy and also indispensable in the treatment of a number of disorders. However, it is contraindicated in conditions of indigestion, vomiting and diarrhea.

Abhyanga can be received from a therapist or self-administered daily to support vibrant skin and a healthy stress response. It is best to do before bathing on an empty stomach in the early morning or before dinner. When applying the oil or fat, the strokes should follow the direction of the body hair, moving down the arms and legs, pausing at all of the joints to massage in a circular motion and giving special emphasis to the massage of the head and feet. As a daily practice, one should massage oil into the body in this way with repeated strokes for at least five minutes to attain thorough results, but of course it can last significantly longer for those who are able. Abhyanga should be followed with some form of fomentation or exposure to heat, such as taking a hot shower or bath, to dilate the pores and allow the healing properties of the fat to penetrate even deeper into the body. When bathing after Abhyanga it is best to avoid soaps and other harsh surfactants, as these will unduly dry the skin, and instead to use herbal wash powders to clean and invigorate the skin without giving stress to the organ's integrity.

External Oleation Therapy is used prior to the Pancha Karma Procedures to calm Vata Dosha and to lubricate and strengthen the body. Additionally, the regular practice of Abhyanga imbues the skin and body with a wonderful softness and elasticity, nourishes the tissues, promotes luster and vibrancy, increases strength, supports healthy circadian rhythms and deep sleep, improves and supports eyesight, reduces and curbs the effects of aging, is useful in mitigating and treating diseases arising from Vata Dosha and supports immunity and resilience to disease.

Svedana: Sudation Therapy

Sudation Therapy describes a wide range of methods that use heat to induce perspiration. The phenomenon of sweating is a natural process that occurs with exercise as well as in warm climates and seasons. This phenomenon is harnessed by Sudation Therapy to relieve stiffness, heaviness, coldness and to relieve specific areas of stagnation and obstruction. This can be accomplished easily even at home by a number of techniques such as Hot Baths, Sitz Baths, Heating Pads, Home Saunas, etc…

The Classical Texts of Ayurveda mention two fundamental types of Sudation Therapy: 1) those which utilize Direct Heat and 2) those which utilize Indirect Heat. Sudation Therapy can be accomplished via Indirect Heat by Exercise, Heavy Blankets, Extra Layers of Warm Clothes, Sunbathing, Hunger, Thirst, Remaining in Closed Quarters, Alcohol, Fear and Anger.

Traditionally in Ayurveda there are 13 methods of Sudation Therapy which utilize Direct Heat, such as bathing in the steam of medicinal herbal teas or decoctions, herbal wraps, pouring streams of warm medicated liquids over the body, massaging the body with hot poultices made from varying substances such as the fresh leaves of medicinal plants, herbal powders, salts, sand and many others. Today the most common method is overwhelmingly the use of Steam Boxes which can be filled with the simple steam of plain water or the steam of various medicinal substances such as herbal decoctions or juices. In some case to treat specific conditions even the steam from substances such as milks or meat broths may be used.

Importantly, unlike Abhyanga, Sudation Therapy shouldn't be employed regularly as overuse can weaken the sensory organs, dry the skin and vitiate the processes of blood production.

Like Oleation Therapy, Sudation Therapy is an important treatment in many disorders, especially those arising from Vata, and is indispensable in preparing one for the Pancha Karma Procedures.

In conjunction with Oleation Therapy which lubricates the bodily channels, gives the body resilience and separates the Doshas from the tissues, Sudation Therapy liquifies the dislodged Doshas, widens the channels and facilitates the movement of the liberated Doshas back to the GI tract for elimination- either upwards through Emetic Therapy or downwards through Purgation Therapy.

To prepare for the Purifying Procedures of Pancha Karma, generally the body is given External Oleation Therapies like Abhyanga after the person has fully digested the fats they have taken internally and then been given Sudation Therapy, most commonly by means of a Sweat Box. However, the specific method of Sudation Therapy should be judged on a case by case basis taking into account constitution, season, environment, strength and the nature of any disorders that may be present. Sudation Therapy usually follows External Oleation Therapy to prepare for the Pancha Karmas but in some cases it may be utilized alone. The duration of the appropriate Sudation Therapy should also vary Patient to Patient, being administered until the person begins to perspire, most commonly for 15-20 minutes.

In addition to preparing the body for the Pancha Karmas,

Sudation Therapy is beneficial in cold climates and seasons, in the treatment of Vata and Vata disorders, to improve hunger, relieve stiffness and increase the mobility of the joints.

PANCHA KARMAS

Purva Karma, the Preparatory Procedures described above, function to strengthen the tissues, remove obstructions in the bodily channels and to collect the Doshas from all over the body into the GI tract. Through close observation and examination, a qualified Ayurvedic Physician will be able to ascertain when this process has reached fruition within the body and therefore determine that the time is ripe to move forward with the Elimination Therapies of Pancha Karma.

At this time, a specific Elimination Therapy will be selected to expel the collected Doshas and waste products through a particular route and bodily opening. Doshas that collects in the stomach are removed through therapeutic vomiting, Vamana. Those which collect in the intestines are expelled through therapeutic purgation, Virechana. Doshas which collect in the head are removed through the nose, Nasya. Doshas collecting in the bladder or colon are removed by medicated enemas, Basti. Doshas collecting throughout the hemopoietic system are liberated relieved through therapeutic bleeding, Rakta Moksha.

Vamana: Emetic Therapy

Vamana literally means 'Vomiting.' Vomiting can transpire under a variety of circumstances such as from motion sickness or food poisoning, using a finger to stimulate the back of the throat, or from drinking salt water. Despite appearances, this Emetic Therapy which Ayurveda employs is quite different from all of the above in its methods and aim. In Ayurveda, Vamana or Emetic Therapy is the method of utilizing specific medicinal substances to expel vitiated Doshas which have been brought to the GI tract from throughout the body via the upward channel of the mouth.

Emetic Therapy purifies the body and is especially useful for treating disorders arising from Kapha[7] and Pitta Doshas such as Rhinitis, Asthma, Skin Disorders, Chronic Cough, Fevers, Indigestion, Nodular Swellings and Allergies. Emetic Therapy is especially useful as a regular treatment for those who are overweight and most efficacious for this purpose when it is performed during the Spring.

Due to the intensive nature of this Purifying Procedure, it is essential that body is properly prepared via Oleation and Sudation Therapies. Usually 5-7 days of Internal Oleation are done in conjunction with External Oleation Therapy and Sudation Therapy as per the Patient's strength, constitution, age, disorders and with consideration for the season and environment.

On the day prior to the Emetic Therapy, a special diet which may consist of Fish or Rice with Yoghurt or Khichadhi made with Urad Dahl is given to increase and liquify the Doshas which have been brought to the GI tract, thereby ensuring their easy expulsion.

On the day of the Emetic Therapy itself the Patient will receive External Oleation and Sudation Therapies and then begin consuming the medicinal substance meant to induce vomiting. These are usually administered in the form of herbal teas and decoctions which have been specifically selected for the Patient and their unique disorders. When properly administered, this method of Emetic Therapy should protect the esophageal lining of the throat from any corrosive

---

[7] Kapha Dosha is composed of the Earth and Water Elements. When imbalanced it creates Poor, Slow Digestion, Excessive Salivation, Laziness and Inertia, Heaviness, Pallor, Coldness, Flaccidity, Breathing Difficulties, Cough and Excessive Sleep.

digestive juices and should draw out the vitiated Kapha and Pitta Doshas effortlessly and with minimal aggravation or discomfort. The herbal teas and decoctions are given continuously until all of the Doshas have been expelled and the proper symptoms of the treatment start to appear such as lightness of the chest, abdomen and body, feelings of relief, clarity of the senses and gentle fatigue.

After the Emetic Therapy, an herbal mouthwash is given and then the medicinal smoke of different herbs is gently inhaled to remove any residual Kapha Dosha that may still be lining the channels from the Emetic Therapy. Then the Patient is encouraged to rest but not to sleep until their hunger returns.

When the digestive fire returns after Emetic Therapy, it is very feeble like a spark that has just been kindled. For this reason, it is extremely important to observe a very specific and regimented diet to slowly rebuild the digestive fire into a powerful flame. This regimented diet is usually observed for 4-5 days.

Emetic Therapy is effective in curing a number of disorders arising from the Doshas and is useful in the prevention of many others. It is traditionally performed as a preventative health measure once a year during the Spring to prevent weight gain, allergies, tendency towards fever, cough/cold and other deficiencies of immunity.

Out of all the Pancha Karma Procedures, Emetic Therapy is simultaneously the one which is most capable of giving rapid and radical results as well as the one most dependent on the compliance of the Patient undergoing the treatment.

To realize the benefits of Emetic Therapy the rules and regulations of its proper administration must be strictly adhered to. Further, the selection of the appropriate Oleation and Sudation Therapies as well as of the herbal preparations to induce Emesis which will be uniquely suitable to a particular person with consideration of environment, season, constitution, disorder, etc… must be overseen by an expert in the field. Thus it is critical that Emetic Therapy and all of the procedures surrounding it are coordinated under the guidance and supervision of a competent Ayurvedic Physician.

Virechana: Purgation Therapy

Many traditional cultures around the world have embraced the routine usage of purgatives. In ancient times in India it was common for each person to take purgatives every six months. Even in the US in places such as Idaho amongst many farming families it was a common practice up until as recently as the 1970s for each member of a family to take castor oil to induce a purge once every summer to stave of the ill effects of the seasonal heat and to maintain health and immunity.

While the seasonal observance of simple purgation by the above methods is surely helpful for eliminating accumulated wastes from the GI tract and strengthening digestion, Virechana, the Purgation Therapy of Ayurveda, has the more profound objective of discharging not only waste products but also the Doshas themselves, thereby eradicating the elements responsible for disease pathogenesis from their root. This form of Purgation Therapy is especially helpful in the treatment of disorders arising from Pitta Dosha such as Jaundice, Skin Disorders, Piles and Hemorrhoids, Digestive Disorders, Asthma, Chronic Fevers, Genital Disorders, Parasites, Blood Disorders and Chronic Toxicity. Generally, Purgation Therapy is contraindicated during Pregnancy, Childhood and in cases of Heart Disease.

To properly execute this Purgation, the body is prepared for

5-7 days utilizing the same techniques employed in Emetic Therapy, namely: Internal and External Oleation Therapy and Sudation Therapy with due regard and differential consideration for the Patient's strength, constitution, age, disease, the environment, season, etc… Again as in the preparation for Emetic Therapy, when the body has been thoroughly lubricated within and without, the Doshas become dislodged from the bodily tissues and collect in the digestive tract for elimination, but in this case via the downward route.

When the above stage has been realized in the body and the Doshas are ready for expulsion there will be a gap of one day from Internal Oleation and on the following morning the appropriate herbal preparations to induce Purgation Therapy are given. However, Purgation Therapy should not be administered in cloudy weather or on days that are very hot or very cold. On the appropriate day the Patient should have a light breakfast of Mung Dahl soon after Sunrise. After sufficient time has been given for the initial stages of digestion (approximately 2 to 2 ½ hours) and the cold of the morning has been relieved by the warmth of the day, the Patient again receives Abhyanga and Sudation Therapy and immediately thereafter consumes the appropriate Purgative Herbal preparation which has been selected by their Physician with due consideration of the nature of their alimentary canal, digestive capacity, age, strength, constitution, etc…. Different herbal preparations can have dramatically different effects on individuals with varying natures in their alimentary canals and digestive capacities and so it is of the utmost importance that this process is overseen by a qualified Physician.

Most purgative herbal preparations will begin to take effect within 2 to 3 hours, stimulating five to twenty rounds of elimination. Initially, the natural wastes and fecal matter will be expelled, then Pitta Dosha in the form of loose stools with varying colors such as yellow, orange, green or red and thereafter Kapha Dosha in the form of mucus. After Kapha has been eliminated the rounds of elimination will cease of their own accord. Prior to the first elimination it is common for the Patient to experience some nausea or digestive discomfort but this is almost always relieved once the elimination begins. Sometimes when there is a great presence of Kapha Dosha or if the Doshas generally have collected more in the space of the stomach rather than in the small intestine the purgative drugs can also stimulate Emesis during the beginning of Purgation as the liberated Doshas will exit the body through the nearest available route.

After taking the purgative herbal preparation, the Patient should abstain from eating and sleeping until the eliminations have finished and they receive further instruction from their Physician. Also they should avoid going outside and all direct exposure to breezes. During this period, it is important that the Patient drink only hot water and use only hot water externally as well to wash hands, etc… After every elimination the Patient should drink at least a sip of hot water and take note of their stool so they can convey the needed information

to their Physician who can assess which Doṣas have been eliminated. In the event that a Patient experiences lingering digestive pain or discomfort even after the eliminations of the Purgation begin, this discomfort is usually easily relieved by the application of a hot water-bag compress. If there is any burning sensation in the anus during elimination from the expulsion of Pitta, the Patient can easily soothe this discomfort by the local application of Ghee.

As the eliminations wind down and the Purgation Therapy draws to a close the Patient should feel lightness throughout the body and especially in the abdominal region. They will feel enthusiasm, great clarity in their senses and like in Emetic Therapy, some fatigue. Also as in Emetic Therapy, when hunger returns the Patient must observe a specific, regimented diet for several days to properly restore the digestive fire.

Without the proper observance and administration of Preparatory Therapies, with improper selection of the purgative herbal preparation with regards to the status of the Patient or with improper management during or after Purgation Therapy, serious complications can occur which can themselves be the cause for a number of disorders. Thus, Purgation Therapy should only ever be done under the guidance and supervision of a qualified Physician.

Basti: Medicated Enema Therapy

Long before the advent of intravenous fluids, the Physicians of Ayurveda administered numerous herbal preparations directly into the anal canal to reach the deep tissues of the body and to manage different acute disorders. This form of treatment is known as Basti in Ayurveda. Though commonly referred to simply as 'Enema Therapy,' Basti Therapy greatly exceeds the understanding and application of enemas as they are employed in the West. Basti Therapy utilizes a wide range of medicinal substances to treat very specific disorders.

Basti literally means 'bladder.' This treatment is called Basti in Ayurveda because in ancient times prior to the invention of catheters and syringes, Physicians used the cleaned and fashioned bladders of animals to administer herbal preparations in this way. Now of course Physicians use equipment such as enema bags or pots with catheters or syringes.

The concept of Basti Therapy most commonly implies the administration of herbal preparations into the colon, however it is also used to describe the administration of herbal preparations through the vagina and urethra. These latter applications are called 'Uttar Basti' in Ayurveda.

Basti Therapy is mostly used for disorders of Vata Dosha. Through Basti Therapy, herbal preparations are absorbed through the large intestine and thereby spread throughout the body into the deepest tissues, pulling Doshas back into the large intestine. The large intestine is the main seat of Vata in the body. Nonetheless, Basti Therapy is often used in the treatment of disorders arising from Pitta and Kapha Doshas as well just by switching the herbal preparations which are used. For Kapha Dosha, Bastis are given using scraping and reducing substances such as Honey and Cow Urine; for Pitta, cooling and soothing substances such as Ghee and Milk.

In the Classical Texts of Ayurveda, it is said that 'Basti Therapy is half of the treatment in all diseases.' On one side of treatment are all of the herbal preparations and treatments of Ayurveda on the other side is Basti Therapy alone, illustrating the unparalleled importance and utility of Basti Therapy within Ayurveda.

 Basti Therapy is divided into two categories: Decoction Enemas and Oil Enemas, which Ayurveda terms as Niruha Basti and Anuvasana Basti respectively. In Decoction Enemas, first a strong Herbal Decoction is prepared and to this honey, salts, herbal powders and different oils or animal fats are added and thoroughly mixed. In the case of oil enemas, just oil or animal fats are employed, sometimes mixed with a small amount of salt.

Decoction Enemas are used in the treatment and management of abdominal disorders, distension, gout, splenic disorders, recurrent fever, runny nose, cough, male and female gynecological disorders and infertility, obstructed feces or urine, scrotal enlargement, urinary stones, amenorrhea and in disorders of the nervous system such as tremors, paralysis, paraplegia, complications of sensory function, etc..

Oil Enemas are used to rebuild strength and stamina in lieu of wasting and debilitation resulting from excessive dryness, fatigue, excessive activity, excessive sex, anxiety, excessive thinking, fractures and injuries and in general convalescence.

Prior to administering Basti Therapy, the body is prepared by External Oleation in the form of Abhyanga and then by Sudation, giving the tissues strength and resilience and widening the internal channels to encourage the Doshas to enter the GI tract. Often is only necessary to apply External Oleation and Sudation to the back, abdomen and thighs to prepare for Basti. This of course will depend upon the individual and disorder.

After the Abhyanga and Sudation, the Patient lays prone with the left leg extended and the right knee bent. A small amount of oil is applied directly to the anus and then a well lubricated catheter is inserted in the direction of the vertebral column to administer the herbal preparations. The fluids are inserted gradually with gentle, uniform pressure and thereafter the Patient rolls over to relax, lying supine with their hips elevated atop a pillow until the urge to release comes.

Decoction Enemas are given immediately after External Oleation and Sudation on an empty stomach. For Oil Enemas, after External Oleation and Sudation the Patient should have a light meal and then receive the Basti. Decoction Enemas are usually expelled along with the Doshas quickly due to the potency of the herbal preparations used. Decoction Enemas cannot be retained for more than 45 minutes and are seldom held for even 10 minutes. The Patient can eat immediately afterwards and must drink only hot water. In the case of Oil Enemas, the Patient should not eat after receiving the Enema until they have expelled it and start to have strong hunger. Oil Enemas are often administered in the evening and held overnight or during the day and held for 3 to 4 hours. In the management of different disorders it is very common for Decoction and Oil Enemas to be given together in a sequence of alternating days, sometimes for an extended period of time up to a month or more.

UTTAR BASTI

As mentioned earlier, Uttar Bastis are Therapeutic Enemas administered via the vaginal or urethral passages. Uttar Bastis use special medicated oils and fats as per the specific disorder to relieve dysfunctions of the urinary system like dysuria, burning, delayed or obstructed micturition, stones, seminal disorders such as poor motility, oligospermia, general reproductive disorders, vaginal disorders and menstrual difficulties. It is especially indicated in infertility and female reproductive disorders.

For women, Uttar Basti is usually preceded by Purgation Therapy or Rectal Basti Therapy as these treatments clear the internal passages and thereby promote the efficacy and potency of Uttar Basti. After completing these cleansing measures, the vaginal passage is further treated by douching with specific herbal decoctions, a practice called Yoni Dhavana in Ayurveda. Thereafter, Uttar Basti is administered by inserting a catheter through the cervical passage, ideally immediately after the cessation of menstruation. This Uttar Basti itself is then followed by the insertion of tampons which have been soaked in medicated oils or fats. These medicated tampons are called as Picchus in Ayurveda. All of these procedures must be performed with great care and stringent hygienic practices by a qualified Physician. When properly executed, Uttar Basti is exceptional in improving the quality and function of the uterus and in treating female reproductive disorders such as ovarian cysts.

Nasya: Errhine Therapy

Ayurveda utilizes virtually all of the bodily orifices to administer herbal preparations and treatments, ie the colon, mouth, ears, eyes and nose. For all disorders above the clavicles and especially for diseases of the head, the nasal passage is the most important route for the administration of herbal preparations. In Ayurveda it is said the nasal passage is the gateway to the head and brain. Thus by administering appropriate herbal preparations via the nasal passage the Doshas and morbid materials collected throughout the head, neck and face are dislodged, scratched out and expelled through the nostrils. This treatment is known as Nasya, or Errhine Therapy.

The overall action of Errhine Therapy can vary greatly as per the medicinal substances that are used. Generally substances such as milk or ghee will be soothing and pacifying for the Doshas and even tonifying, while substance such as medicated smoke, herbal powders and strong herbal decoctions will be more purifying.

The ideal seasonal times to perform Errhine Therapy are just before rainy seasons, during early Autumn and immediately before Spring. However as per necessity, Errhine Therapy can be administered at almost any time by creating an opportune environment in which it is neither too hot nor too cold, neither too dry nor too moist.

In the process of administering Errhine Therapy first the head, face and neck are massaged thoroughly with appropriate oily substances. Then these same parts are given Sudation Therapy though localized steam. The medicinal substance is brought to a lukewarm temperature and with the Patient lying down, the head is tilted back, the tip of the nose is raised and the substance is delivered into the nasal passages drop by drop. The head is gently massaged to encourage the herbal preparation's dispersion and absorption while the Patient relaxes, avoiding speech, anger, laughing, sneezing and shaking. To calm and ground the nervous system, the hands and feet are also gently massaged at this time.

When the action of the herbal preparations reach a climax, the Patient sits up and the Doshas, especially Kapha, begin to leave the head through the nasal passages along with the herbal preparations that were used. It is very important that the Patient makes an effort not to swallow but rather to spit out any and all discharge. Even if the herbal preparation or discharge enters the oropharynx it should be spat out rather than swallowed as it is mixed with Doshas which should not be allowed to re-enter circulation.

The above method of administering Errhine Therapy is useful in the treatment of headaches, neck stiffness and disorders of the cervical vertebrae, hoarseness of voice, vision and ocular disorders, tonsillitis, rhinitis, facial paralysis, disorders of the mouth and especially TMJ and lockjaw. However, given the intensive nature of this treatment, it is contraindicated after eating, after drinking, during indigestion, when there is strong hunger, while fasting, after bathing, when experiencing fatigue, after coitus, after exercise, during fever, rhinitis, pregnancy, post-partum, in cases of poisoning and after having undergone Emetic, Purgation or Basti Therapy.

As a far less intensive and restrictive practice, Ayurveda encourages the regular application of gentle Errhine Therapy, Pratimarsha Nasya, in which just two drops of oil or ghee are inserted into each nostril. This form of Errhine Therapy can be done during any season and at any age, with a number of opportunities throughout the day such as after rising, brushing the teeth, gargling or instilling eye drops, before going out, after exercise or coitus, after walking, urination, defecation and after meals. As a regular practice, this gentle Errhine Therapy gives strength and robustness to the face, neck, head, chest and shoulders, supports cognitive and sensory function and tonifies the brain and sense organs.

Errhine Therapy offers great and unique remedial potential in the modern environment of stress, tension, competition and perpetual sensory and cognitive strain by imbuing the brain and sense organs with greater strength, resilience and adaptive capacity.

Rakta Mokshana: Therapeutic Bleeding

Rakta Mokshana, which literally means the release or liberation of blood, is an ancient practice of removing vitiated blood from the body. The practice of Therapeutic Bleeding can be observed in a variety of ancient and modern cultures from across the globe such as amongst the ancient Maya, the Hebraic Tribes of Israel, Greek and Roman Civilizations, the Islamic cultures of the Middle East and even in contemporary Native American Tribes.

In Ayurveda, Therapeutic Bleeding can be accomplished surgically through venesection or by parasurgical means such as the application of leeches. Therapeutic Bleeding is considered to be a proper Shodhana or purifying treatment in the context of Ayurveda, wherein vitiated blood carrying

toxins and Doṣas is removed from the body. While Emetic Therapy is considered to be the most efficacious in the treatment of Kapha Dosha, Purgation Therapy for Pitta and Basti Therapy for Vata, Therapeutic Bleeding is the therapy to be employed when the blood itself has become vitiated, carrying any one or even all three Doshas throughout the body to corrupt the deeper tissues. Such a circumstance is often revealed when an individual's symptoms are not relieved by either heating or cooling therapies nor by oleating or drying therapies.

The quality of the blood becomes corrupted from the regular intake of hot and spicy food, excessive salt, yoghurt and other fermented foods, wine, day napping, excessive walking or exertion in hot climates and emotions such as anger, sadness and fear.

As the blood becomes vitiated, the Doshas and toxins present within it become more superficial as the body's inherent intelligence yearns for their elimination. Thus, during Therapeutic Bleeding it is this vitiated blood which is the first to be released. In the case of venesection, generally only 100-120ml is taken while in parasurgical methods such as leech application, scratching or using suction even less is taken, approximately 10-20ml. This removal of vitiated blood directly stimulates the production of pure, fresh, healthy blood, which replaces the volume of the blood lost within 48 hours.

Autumn is the ideal time to perform Therapeutic Bleeding as it is neither too hot nor too cold and the skies tend to be clear, but when necessary it can also be performed in cooler seasons during mid day when it is warmest or during hot seasons during the early morning when there is some coolness.

To prepare for Therapeutic Bleeding generally a Patient will consume Mahatiktaka Ghrta, an ancient recipe of herbalized, bitter ghee for 5 to 7 days, but of course this will vary as per circumstances. So too will the decision of whether to go for venesection or to employ one of the parasurgical methods of Therapeutic Bleeding such as the application of leeches or suction using horns or cupping techniques.

Venesection is indicated in cases where all of the blood in circulation is vitiated giving rise to systemic disorders. If blood is observed to be impure in a single place it can be released by different methods of scratching, which is also indicated generally for the management of Kapha, especially by using bitter gourd to make the scratches. In disorders of Vata and when the impurities are lodged deep below the surface of the skin, they are best released by suction methods such as cupping. When there is only a local disturbance or in disorders of Pitta, leeches are indicated.

The practice of employing leeches for Therapeutic Bleeding is currently experiencing a resurgence even in Western Allopathic medicine. When leeches are applied to an affected area, they puncture the skin and begin to draw out vitiated blood. Hirudin present in their saliva inhibits clotting factors to prevent clots while they are drawing blood. Once they have become satiated they will release of their own accord or the Physician may determine to remove them prior to this by using turmeric or salt to force them to detach. The site of their bite may remain for a few days after the treatment, but this process is relatively painless and devoid of discomfort, making it fit even for children and the elderly.

In modern medical practice leeches are destroyed after their application but in Ayurveda leeches are preserved as a single leech can be employed for years. To this end, after each application the leeches are given turmeric, forcing them to vomit all of the vitiated blood they have drawn, and then they are massaged with oil and rock salt. After this process and 10 days of rest they can be reused, though they are again soaked in turmeric water for 30-45 minutes before applications and a sterilizing measure.

After Therapeutic Bleeding individuals should resort to light, soupy foods which are easy to digest until their digestive strength is restored, giving great care to avoid excessively hot, cold, heavy and stale foods. Anger, day napping and exposure to heat should also be avoided after Therapeutic Bleeding.

Therapeutic Bleeding is particularly useful in the treatment of skin problems, splenomegaly, jaundice, piles, pimples, vision and ocular disorders, hypertension, abscesses, liver disorders, headaches, tendency towards having bloody noses or blood mixed in the urine or stool and in joint disorders. In joint disorders particularly, Therapeutic Bleeding can bring near instantaneous relief. It is encouraged by Ayurveda during Autumn even for the healthy person to maintain pure, healthy blood. It is contraindicated during pregnancy, chronic fatigue and when there is swelling throughout the body.

Therapeutic Bleeding is a simple but profoundly effective treatment. Like Basti Therapy, Ayurveda considers it to be half of the treatment for a number of disorders.

PASHCHAT KARMA:
CARE DURING AND AFTER PANCHA KARMA

The purifying therapies of Ayurveda which have been described thus far require great care and attention as well as sufficient time, a suitable environment and supervision by a qualified Physician to yield forth their healing potentials and to bar the production of any ill effects.

Having undergone such thorough and deep reaching therapies, Patients find their tissues enlivened and renewed but also fragile and impressionable to environmental circumstances. Thus there is a great need for support and supervision after undergoing any of the Pancha Karma therapies. Ayurveda describes the post-procedural patient as being like an unhatched egg which must be handled with great care, attention, delicacy, love and affection as they hatch into renewed health and vitality. A similar example is given of a vessel holding oil, which must be carried carefully with equipoise and grace so as not to spill. Thus it is incumbent upon the Physician to guide and watch over the Patients under their care with the same attention and diligence found in a shepherd overseeing his or her flock.

The post-procedural observances which protect and restore the Patient after undergoing any of the Pancha Karmas fundamentally consist of a specific and graduated diet and behavioral restrictions.

SAMSARJAN KRAMA: GRADUATED DIET

In the wake of Pancha Karma procedures and also of acute illnesses such as fever, the digestive fire becomes weak and fragile as the body diverts its energy resources to healing and eliminatory functions. Thus, the tiny spark of the digestive fire has to be kindled and rebuilt step-by-step through a graduated diet just as a fire is built first with kindling material, then leaves and small twigs proceeding to larger sticks and finally logs. During this process, the consistency and amount of food is increased slowly, step-by-step until the digestive fire is capable to return to a normal diet.

Further, with a substantial amount of the Doshas eliminated, the body is like a freshly tilled and weeded plot of soil, waiting to manifest any number of potentials. However, the garden that is to grow is totally dependent upon the first seeds sown and so this process of rebuilding the fire uses the following very specific recipes which increase in density one to the next:

- **Peya- Rice Broth:** 1 part of roasted rice is well cooked in 14 parts of water on low heat to create a broth. To this a small amount of cumin and salt can be added for taste and to stimulate digestion. Overall this Rice Broth is very light and helps to slowly build up the digestive fire while providing a basic nourishment to the tissues and encouraging the gentle elimination of any residual Doshas.
- **Vilepi- Rice Porridge:** this is similar to the above preparation but it is of a slightly thicker consistency. It has the same general properties but begins to imbue the body with more strength.
- **Yusha- Lentil Broth:** this recipe is also prepared in the same way as the above two but uses lentils in place of rice, most commonly mung beans.
- **Mamsa Rasa- Meat Broth:** small pieces of meat such as chicken, goat or beef are first sautéed in ghee and then boiled with ample water to prepare a light but invigorating soup. This broth is both stabilizing

and greatly restorative to the tissues, giving strength, vigor and a much stronger appetite.
- **Khichari:** this is a porridge like substance prepared by cooking well washed rice and mung beans (or other lentils) together until they reach a thick consistency. It is the final and heaviest item in the graduated diet before returning to normal foods.

The length of time required for observing this graduated diet will vary by the intensity of the purifying therapies and the amount of Doshas which were eliminated. If the therapy proved to be deeply purifying with ample discharge of Dosha then this graduated diet should be drawn out for seven days. If the therapy was quite mild with only a small amount of Dosha eliminated then even three days may be sufficient, while for medium intensity and medium elimination five days is indicated. Ultimately however it is when the digestive fire proves that it is burning bright and strong enough to transform whatever food stuffs and experiences it meets that the graduated diet should be relinquished.

BEHAVIORAL RESTRICTIONS

In addition to observing a graduated diet, after Pancha Karma Therapies Patients must adhere to certain Do's and Don'ts in their day to day activities and lifestyles to truly reap the benefits of the treatments.

- As in Internal Oleation Therapy, Patients should only use warm water, both for drinking and for bathing.
- Excessively cold or hot things and environments generally should be avoided.
- Upon completion of the graduated diet, food articles which are antagonistic to the constitution or

disorders of a Patient should be strictly avoided as per the instructions of their Physician.

- Food should be taken only when there is ample hunger and the previous meal has been digested.
- Loud and excessive speaking expend a surprising amount of energy and also can create disturbance in the mind. Thus, they should be avoided so as to utilize the same energy for restorative purposes.
- Situations which stimulate intense emotions, especially Anger and Sorrow, should be avoided for as long as possible to allow both mind and body to settle and gain strength.
- Intense physical activity such as exercise and even undue walking up and down stairs should be put off until the body is strong and energized.
- The body should not be constrained or confined after treatment. Long travel, sleeping in cars or planes or sitting continuously for an extended period in one position even for meditation should be avoided.
- Napping and sleeping during the day should be avoided as this creates obstruction in the bodily channels and increases Kapha Dosha.
- Staying up late and not getting sufficient sleep at night should also be avoided as this does just the opposite, reducing Kapha, increasing Vata and creating dryness in the body.
- Sex should be avoided until the body has returned to normal strength.
- None of the body's natural urges such as the urge for urination, defecation, eructation, laughing, yawning, etc… should be forced or withheld, especially so the urges for defecation and urination.

Conclusion

Before the traumas and travails of life, should illnesses develop within us we can feel as though we are buried and constricted beneath our circumstances and woes. Upon finding effective treatment, as healing begins, it is a most delicate and vulnerable process. The life breath begins to break through the amassed earth to behold the sky like a tender sprout shooting forth from the seeds of our hearts.

This journey requires great care, attention and respect. It cannot be packaged. It cannot be streamlined or systematized or depersonalized. It takes time. It takes relationship. It takes knowledge and skill in practice. Sprouts arise by the dictate of the seasons. Should the weather turn, they must be protected by the wise gardener, the capable Physician. As the leaves unfurl, specific nutrients should be sowed into the soil to promote their growth and luster. With growth comes new experience and challenge. Pruning may be in order.

Thus, healing is an ever dynamic process. It is the journey to realize equipoise and rhythm amidst the revolving cycles of life, learning to dance with the ebb and flow of the tides. There is rarely if ever a moment of calm or stillness as the tides ebb and flow. So too there is rarely if ever a moment or activity in life that is totally free from or beyond the Doshas. Even as the tides surge forth, there are inevitable excitations of Doshas, of discomfort and aggravation. But, barring obstruction, that which surges forth also recedes back into the ocean. Symptoms arise only to dissipate. Doshas well forth and permeate the body, but once vitiating factors are removed, they return to their sources and their presence in the tissues is replaced by strength and vitality. By taking proper and judicious resort to profound treatments such as those of Pancha Karma and through deference and adherence

to nature's wisdom, may all beings emerge from the toss of
the tides and come to behold ever with wonder the majesty of
life and creation.

ABOUT THE AUTHORS

VAIDYA VARSHA GALGALI (MD AYU)

In lieu of completing her MD from the prestigious Gujarat Ayurved University in Jamnagar, where she graduated first in her class, Vaidya Varsha Galgali has maintained a busy clinical practice in Pune, India, serving thousands of patients for the last 19 years. Her practice specializes in the procedures of Pancha Karma.

Vaidya Varsha began her study of Ayurveda at Tilak Vidyapeeth, after which she completed her BAMS through Babsahed Abedkar Marathwada University where she was a Gold Medal winner. Ever beholden of a strong academic capacity, in the space beyond her clinical practice Vaidya Varsha maintains an academic presence as well. She was a lecturer at Wagholi college from 2000-2003 and is currently on the teaching faculty of Ayurveda College Akurdi and has been an instructor for the MUHS Post Graduate Diploma Course in Pancha Karma operated by Punarvasu Ayurveda Prabodhini for more than 10 years.

Beyond instruction, Vaidya Varsha is also an established researcher. She worked for 3 ½ years as a researcher in the Cancer Research Project at Wagholi, spent 2 years pursuing post graduate research at GUA in Jamnagar and currently works as a research guide for post graduate students.

KASHYAPA FISHER

Kashyapa began his study of Yoga, Ayurveda and Vedic Culture in 2008 while living in India for four years in a monastic setting. He began formal training in Ayurveda in 2013, completing the US-based Ayurvedic Studies Program with Dr Lad at the Ayurvedic Institute. Kashyapa thereafter returned to India for an intensive and classical education in the clinical application of Ayurveda with his primary mentors, Vaidyas Shreerang and Varsha Galgali (MD Ayu) of Arogyasarathi Cikitsalaya in Pune, India who continue to guide him in the practice of authentic Ayurveda to this day.

Additionally, Kashyapa studied Sanskrit in Deccan College, Pune and has been trained and certified in Massage Therapy, Naturopathy, Emergency Medicine, Functional Allopathy and

Keraliya techniques of Pancha Karma. Kashyapa served on the teaching faculty for The Ayurvedic Institute's ASP1 & 2 Programs in Albuquerque, New Mexico from 2015-2017, where he also served as a Professional Clinician and Clinic Supervisor. He teaches and lectures throughout the US and India and currently maintains a clinical practice in Albuquerque, New Mexico and online, offering Ayurvedic Consulting and traditional Pancha Karma.

www.ingramcontent.com/pod-product-compliance
Lightning Source LLC
Chambersburg PA
CBHW072301260726
48658CB00002BA/904